39 REASONS
HEALING IS YOURS

Healing Scriptures That **Beat Sickness to Death**

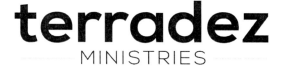

TABLE OF CONTENTS

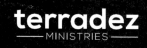

Jesus bore **every** sickness and disease on the cross so that you could live a healed life. God wants you to be healed and whole, in both your soul and your physical body!

It has been said that Jesus took 39 stripes for 39 different root causes of disease. Therefore, we compiled a list of 39 healing scriptures as a resource that will bring you revelation regarding the healing Jesus provided at the cross.

As you apply the Word of God to your life, these healing scriptures will beat sickness to death!

BULLET POINTS

Each of these healing scriptures contains bullet points below to bring out key themes from the verse. Our intention in adding these notes is to help you gain insight into these scriptures, rather than just a superficial glance at a list. However, God has so much more for you than we can fit inside the pages of this booklet! We encourage you to study them for yourself and allow the Holy Spirit to give you revelation regarding how each one applies to your unique situation.

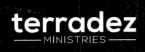
MAKE IT YOUR OWN

The final bullet point of each scripture contains a related prayer and way to speak them over your life. As you grow in your relationship with the Lord, it will become more and more natural for you to take the Word, pray it, and confess it. To help those who are just beginning this journey with God, we have added the "Make It Your Own" section as a way to teach how to begin using the Word in your everyday life!

MEDITATE AND CONFESS

We believe that as you meditate on and confess these healing scriptures over yourself, your faith will rise. These scriptures prove that it is always God's will for you to live in physical health and emotional wholeness. As you develop a revelation of these truths, you will be empowered to receive the healing Jesus already provided!

⁴ Surely He has borne our griefs And carried our sorrows; Yet we esteemed Him stricken, Smitten by God, and afflicted. ⁵ But He was wounded for our transgressions He was bruised for our iniquities; The chastisement for our peace was upon Him. And by His stripes we are healed.

- The word for "griefs" is the Hebrew word *choli,* which means sickness.

- The word for "sorrows" is the Hebrew word *makob,* which means pain. This certainly applies to both physical and emotional pain.

- The word for "healed" is the Hebrew word *raphe,* which means to heal, to mend, to cure, to make whole.

- Jesus bore all of our sickness and pain on the cross, so that by the scourging He took on our behalf, we could be made completely well, both physically and emotionally.

MAKE IT YOUR OWN:

Thank You, Jesus, for taking all sickness and pain on the cross for me. You became sick, so that I could be healed! I receive by faith the physical health and emotional wholeness that You bought for me when You took stripes on your back and died on the cross.

Who Himself bore our sins in His own body on the tree, that we, having died to sins, might live for righteousness—by whose stripes you were healed.

- When Jesus died on the cross, He became sin for us so that we would be made the righteousness of God in Him (2 Corinthians 5:21).
- In the same way, Jesus took stripes and was beaten for our healing as well!

MAKE IT OWN:

Thank You, Jesus, that just like You became sin for me so that I could die to sin and be made alive to righteousness, by Your stripes I was healed as well. I believe that healing is past tense: I was healed by Your stripes! Since I *was* healed, I *am* healed, in Jesus' name.

So when Jesus had received the sour wine, He said, "It is finished!" And bowing His head, He gave up His spirit.

- When Jesus died, the work He had been sent to accomplish was complete.

- He doesn't ever have to die again for your salvation, and He doesn't have to die again for your physical healing. It was all done when He died on the cross!

MAKE IT YOUR OWN:

Lord, I agree with You: It is finished! My salvation was finished at the cross, and my healing was finished at the cross, too. This sickness is finished, in Jesus' name!

² Bless the Lord, O my soul; And all that is within me, bless His holy name! Bless the Lord, O my soul, And forget not all His benefits: ³ Who forgives all your iniquities, Who heals all your diseases, ⁴ Who redeems your life from destruction, Who crowns you with lovingkindness and tender mercies, ⁵ Who satisfies your mouth with good things, So that your youth is renewed like the eagle's.

- Just like David, who wrote this Psalm, we have to remind ourselves to remember the benefits that come from our faith in Jesus.

- These benefits include forgiveness of all sins and healing of all diseases!

- Notice that renewed youth is another benefit of our relationship with God.

MAKE IT YOUR OWN:

Lord, I'm not going to forget the benefits that are part of my relationship with You! Thank You for forgiving all of my sins, healing all of my diseases, redeeming my life from destruction, and crowning me with lovingkindness and tender mercies. Thank You, Lord, for satisfying my mouth with good things. My youth is renewed!

⁹ Because you have made the Lord, who is my refuge, Even the Most High, your dwelling place, ¹⁰ No evil shall befall you, Nor shall any plague come near your dwelling... ¹⁴ "Because he has set his love upon Me, therefore I will deliver him; I will set him on high, because he has known My name. ¹⁵ He shall call upon Me, and I will answer him; I will be with him in trouble; I will deliver him and honor him. ¹⁶ With long life I will satisfy him, And show him My salvation."

○ Whenever you find yourself under attack, you can call out to the Lord and He WILL deliver you, every single time!

○ Notice that these benefits of protection, health, deliverance, long life, and salvation are all based on personal relationship with the Lord.

○ NO evil shall befall you and NO plague is allowed entrance to your dwelling. These are benefits that you can claim for yourself and walk in by faith.

MAKE IT YOUR OWN:

Lord, You are my refuge, and I dwell in You! No evil shall befall me, and no plague can come near my dwelling, neither my house nor my body. You always answer me. You are with me in trouble, and you deliver me. You satisfy me with long life!

The thief does not come except to steal, and to kill, and to destroy. I have come that they may have life, and that they may have it more abundantly.

- The word for "abundantly" is the Greek word *perissos*, which means "more, greater, excessive, exceedingly, vehemently".

- This abundant life surpasses the expected limit!

- The word for "thief" is the Greek word *kleptés*, which makes the distinction between a thief who steals by stealth, rather than through violence.

- The enemy is a subtle thief, so we need to be aware of his tricks of deception: i.e. that God has caused your sickness, or the Word won't work for you, or this sickness is "normal".

MAKE IT YOUR OWN:

I believe that Jesus came so that I would live an abundant life! I refuse to settle for the lies of the thief in my life. I reject those lies and I receive the abundant life that Jesus died for me to have! Rather than just a normal life, I live the abundant life: in righteousness, divine health and wholeness, and financial provision.

I shall not die, but live, And declare the works of the Lord.

- Perhaps your physical challenge isn't terminal. Maybe it's chronic pain, or a skin condition, or a digestive issue, but it isn't an actual death sentence.

- However, anything less than the abundant life Jesus died for you to have is "death" to some degree.

- When you live the abundant life that Jesus died for you to live, you are a living, breathing, walking billboard of the works of God!

MAKE IT YOUR OWN:

I will not die! I will live an abundant life, and I will declare the works of the Lord!

What do you conspire against the Lord? He will make an utter end of it. Affliction will not rise up a second time.

○ Sometimes we receive a healing from the Lord, but lying symptoms try to come to convince us, "You thought you were healed, but it was only temporary relief. You aren't *really* healed!"

○ That is a lie! That attempt of sickness to come back on your body is a conspiracy against the Lord. Your body is the temple of the Holy Spirit, and it is trying to sneak back in.

○ Yet, the Word says that this affliction cannot come a second time!

MAKE IT YOUR OWN:

By the stripes of Jesus, I was healed! I reject these symptoms, and I command them to leave my body. This sickness cannot come back a second time, in Jesus' name.

'For I will restore health to you And heal you of your wounds,' says the Lord...

- What an incredible promise! You can receive this promise for yourself right now, by faith, because of what Jesus did for you at the cross.

- This verse can apply to any situation that has attacked your body, even injury due to an accident.

- For example: Carlie broke her ankle in a field one day, but she jumped up and declared her healing and ran home. By the time she got back to the house, her ankle was healed! He will heal you of your wounds!

MAKE IT YOUR OWN:

Father God, I thank You for Your promise to me that you will restore my health and heal my wounds! Thank You, Jesus, for dying on the cross so that I can claim this promise for myself. Health, be restored, and wounds, you are healed, in Jesus' name!

20 My son, give attention to my words; Incline your ear to my sayings. 21 Do not let them depart from your eyes; Keep them in the midst of your heart; 22 For they are life to those who find them, And health to all their flesh. 23 Keep your heart with all diligence, For out of it spring the issues of life.

- The Bible is full of God's words, His sayings. For us to fully live in His promises, we have to keep ourselves in His Word.

- The word "keep" means to keep, watch, or preserve. This basically means to guard the Word of God that has been planted in your heart. The Word should be a primary focus in your life, which you give great weight to and put your trust in.

- The Scriptures themselves will bring life and health to you!

- Take care for the things that you allow into your heart (through what you see, hear, read, and speak).

MAKE IT YOUR OWN:

Lord, I place Your Word in high priority in my life. I follow the wisdom that I find in it, and I focus on it throughout my day. Your Word is life to me, and brings health to my flesh! Holy Spirit, thank You for giving me the wisdom and ability I need to guard my heart diligently, so that life and strength flow into me, from the inside, every day.

But if the Spirit of Him who raised Jesus from the dead dwells in you, He who raised Christ from the dead will also give life to your mortal bodies through His Spirit who dwells in you.

○ Are you born again? If you are, then the Spirit who raised Jesus from the dead dwells inside of you!

○ The life of the Spirit of God in you continuously releases life into your physical body!

○ That life includes the energy and ability to accomplish what is set before you every single day.

MAKE IT YOUR OWN:

Thank You, Lord, for giving me the Holy Spirit! Your Spirit releases Your power into my physical, mortal body, so sickness, disease, and fatigue—anything that is contrary to abundant life—cannot stay in me. Your power is pushing out every trespasser, in Jesus' name. Thank You for giving me Your life!

14 *Is anyone among you sick? Let him call for the elders of the church, and let them pray over him, anointing him with oil in the name of the Lord.* **15** *And the prayer of faith will save the sick, and the Lord will raise him up. And if he has committed sins, he will be forgiven.* **16** *Confess your trespasses to one another, and pray for one another, that you may be healed. The effective, fervent prayer of a righteous man avails much.*

- If you are sick, get some like-minded believers to agree with you for your healing.

- There is power for healing in confessing your sin to other believers. Hiding sin actually gives that sin power. When you confess it, it releases the power of sin over you so that you can be healed: not only physically, but *set free from that sin as well*.

- As a born-again believer, you have already been made righteous! (2 Corinthians 5:21). Your righteousness, and therefore the effectiveness of your prayers, is not based on your actions. It is based on your faith in Jesus! As a believer, your prayers are POWERFUL and EFFECTIVE!

MAKE IT YOUR OWN:

Father, I thank You that my prayers are powerful and effective, because I am the righteousness of God in Christ Jesus! I know that as I pray faith-filled prayers, the sick are saved!

14 Now this is the confidence that we have in Him, that if we ask anything according to His will, He hears us. *15* And if we know that He hears us, whatever we ask, we know that we have the petitions that we have asked of Him.

- You cannot pray a prayer of faith unless you know the will of God.

- The most common question regarding this verse is, "How do we know what God's will is, so that we can pray according to His will?"

- God's will is found in His Word! Are you praying for healing? That's His will! Are you praying for increase so that you are able to give more into the Kingdom of God and be a living advertisement of His goodness? That's His will! Are you praying for a godly spouse who will partner with you in serving the Lord? That's His will!

- The word "anything" in this verse means just that: ANYTHING! You can have boldness that when you pray, God is sending the answer.

MAKE IT YOUR OWN:

Thank You, Lord, for revealing Your will to me in Your Word. Your will for me is always for good, so I know that when I pray regarding those good things, You hear me, and You have granted me what I have asked!

¹⁷ And these signs will follow those who believe: In My name they will cast out demons; they will speak with new tongues; ¹⁸ they will take up serpents; and if they drink anything deadly, it will by no means hurt them; they will lay hands on the sick, and they will recover.

- This scripture is not directed at a small group of elites! The qualification is that these signs will follow ***those who believe!***

- If you believe in what Jesus has told you through the Word, then ***you*** qualify to do all of these things, including laying hands on the sick and seeing them recover.

- A little note on this scripture, regarding the first part of verse 18: Don't go out playing with venomous snakes and intentionally drinking poison! This is talking about if something comes against you, it will not harm you. But don't "tempt the Lord", which is how Jesus responded to the devil when He tempted Him to jump off the top of the temple in Matthew 4:5-7.

- However, when Paul was bitten by a viper, he shook it off into the fire and was not harmed (Acts 28:3-5). That is the kind of thing this verse is referring to. You can trust God that when something tries to harm you, it can't succeed because you are protected!

MAKE IT YOUR OWN:

I am a believer! Signs and wonders follow me. I can cast out demons, speak in new tongues, nothing can harm me, and when I lay hands on the sick, they will recover! Thank You, Jesus, for giving me the authority to impact the world around me with Your power.

Behold, I give you the authority to trample on serpents and scorpions, and over all the power of the enemy, **and nothing shall by any means hurt you.**

- Read this verse again. And again. Maybe one more time, just to be sure!

- Jesus has given you authority over ALL the power of the enemy. Not just sometimes, or a little bit. ALL AUTHORITY OVER THE ENEMY, ALL THE TIME!

- He said, "**Nothing** shall by **any** means hurt you." NOTHING. By ANY means!

MAKE IT YOUR OWN:

I believe in Jesus. I believe in the power and authority that He has given me over all the power of the enemy, and that nothing shall by any means hurt me! I command any demonic spirit causing sickness to leave my body/_____'s body, in Jesus' name! Thank You, Lord, that I have Your authority and power, that I am protected and anointed, and for revealing these truths to me.

He sent them to preach the kingdom of God and to heal the sick.

o Who was "them" in this verse? In Luke 9:2, Jesus sent out the twelve to preach the kingdom of God and heal the sick.

o However, it didn't stop with the twelve! In Luke 10:1, 9 it says, *"1 After these things the Lord appointed seventy others also, and sent them two by two... 9 "And heal the sick there, and say to them, 'The kingdom of God has come near to you.'"*

o If you hear anyone say that signs and wonders stopped with the disciples, you have to ask, "Which ones?" These verses are for all of us—for all who believe.

MAKE IT YOUR OWN:

I am anointed. Jesus has sent me to preach the kingdom of God and heal the sick!

21 *So Jesus answered and said to them, "Assuredly, I say to you, if you have faith and do not doubt, you will not only do what was done to the fig tree, but also if you say to this mountain, 'Be removed and be cast into the sea,' it will be done.* **22** *And whatever things you ask in prayer, believing, you will receive."*

- The word for "whatever things" in this verse was originally "as many as all things" which are the words *hosa* and *pas*. *Hosa* means "how much, how many, how great, as great as, as much". *Pas* means "all, the whole, every kind of".

- Jesus is saying that if you believe, you will receive every single thing you pray for!

- Jesus is also very intentional here to tell us that we have authority to command every challenge in our lives to be removed!

MAKE IT YOUR OWN:

Jesus gave me authority over the mountains that are in my way. I command this mountain to move, in the name of Jesus! Lord, I thank You that I can ask boldly in prayer and know that I will receive what I have prayed for. I know that when I pray, it is finished!

Jesus said to him, "If you can believe, all things are possible to him who believes."

○ Romans 12:3 says that *"God hath dealt to every man the measure of faith"* (KJV). Each believer has been given faith to believe!

○ Galatians 2:20 says, *"I am crucified with Christ: nevertheless I live; yet not I, but Christ liveth in me: and the life which I now live in the flesh I live by the faith of the Son of God, who loved me, and gave himself for me."*

○ You have the faith of Jesus inside of you, so **you can believe!** Therefore, all things are possible.

MAKE IT YOUR OWN:

Lord, thank You for giving me the faith to believe You for anything I need. I have the faith of Jesus on the inside of me, and I can believe! There is nothing that is impossible for me. I believe that (insert the end result you are believing for) and I receive it by faith right now, in Jesus' name!

22 So Jesus answered and said to them, "Have faith in God. **23** For assuredly, I say to you, whoever says to this mountain, 'Be removed and be cast into the sea,' and does not doubt in his heart, but believes that those things he says will be done, he will have whatever he says. **24** Therefore I say to you, whatever things you ask when you pray, believe that you receive them, and you will have them.

- This verse is the parallel verse to Matthew 21:21-22. However, this verse gives even more clarity to how this principle works.

- Even though you are taking your authority and speaking to the mountain, it is still GOD in whom you are placing your faith, not in your own ability. Keep your faith in Him, not in whether you say or do everything perfectly. It is easy to doubt when you are looking at yourself. Instead, have faith in God, and there will not be room for doubt in your heart.

- When you pray, believe that you receive. If you have received something by faith, even if it is not yet in your hands, you don't keep asking for it. The answer has already been given, and you have already received it. When you believe that you receive, then you will have it!

MAKE IT YOUR OWN:

Lord, I have faith in You! I command this mountain in my life to move, in Jesus' name! Father, I ask
_____. I believe that You have granted to me what I have asked of you, and I receive it right now by faith, in Jesus' name! I thank You that it is finished, and I give You all the glory for it!

But Jesus looked at them and said, "With men it is impossible, but not with God; for with God all things are possible."

- Have you or someone you love been diagnosed with an "incurable" disease? Humanity may not have a cure, but God does!

- Are you on a fixed income and think that there's no way for you to increase? In the natural, it may look impossible, but God can provide in ways you would never expect!

- Jesus healed the incurable, and provided more than enough when it seemed impossible. He loves performing the "impossible" because it gives Him glory!

MAKE IT YOUR OWN:

Lord, I am not putting my trust in what man says is possible or not. I put my trust in Your Word, which says that all things are possible with You. I am excited to see how You are going to turn this "impossible" situation around! It doesn't even matter if I know how, because I know that You fulfill Your promises! (See Hebrews 10:23, page 31).

Blessed is she who believed, for there will be a fulfillment of those things which were told her from the Lord.

○ This verse is referring to Mary, the mother of Jesus. She was told by the angel Gabriel that she would have a baby and believed every word that was spoken to her by God.

○ Mary was blessed because she believed!

○ Mary also received what God had promised her because of her faith. She said, "Let it be to me according to your word" (Luke 1:38).

MAKE IT YOUR OWN:

Lord, I believe what You have said to me through Your Word, specifically that by the stripes of Jesus, I was healed! I am blessed because I believe that God will do everything He has promised me. Let it be to me according to Your Word, in Jesus' name!

Let us hold fast the confession of our hope without wavering, for He who promised is faithful.

- Notice how the emphasis in this verse is not on our hope, but on the faithfulness of God.

- God is always faithful to fulfill every single promise He has made.

- Don't waver! Keep speaking the Word of God (these healing scriptures) over yourself. Do not quit, because God is faithful!

MAKE IT YOUR OWN:

I will not waver in the confession of my hope in the Lord! My God is faithful, and He always fulfills the promises He has made to me in His Word.

Then the Lord said to me, "You have seen well, for I am ready to perform My word."

○ The Lord is ready to perform His Word! He isn't twiddling His thumbs, waiting for just the right moment. He is ready NOW!

○ If there is a delay in receiving from God, it isn't on His part. We are dealing with a fallen world, surrounded by imperfect people, including ourselves.

○ Trust God. He is ready, willing and able to perform His Word in your life! Pray that God will take care of any hindrances, be they other people, the enemy, or even something going on in your own heart.

MAKE IT YOUR OWN:

Lord, I thank You that You are ready to perform your Word! You want me healed and whole even more than I want it for myself. Holy Spirit, if there are any hindrances, show me what they are and how to take authority over them. Give me Your wisdom in this situation (James 1:5). I trust that if there is something I don't know that I need to, You will tell me! Then You will also enable me to take any necessary action.

²⁰ He sent His word and healed them, And delivered them from their destructions. ²¹ Oh, that men would give thanks to the Lord for His goodness, And for His wonderful works to the children of men!

- God sent His Word to heal you and deliver you from all of your destructions. The Word isn't just the Bible: it is Jesus Himself! (See John 1:14, page 35).

- As you are standing in faith for your healing, or any challenge you may be facing, give thanks to the Lord! Thank Him for healing you, thank Him for every good thing in your life. It is a really good practice to write down at **least** one thing you are thankful for every day.

- 1 Thessalonians 5:18 tells us that it is God's will for us to give thanks in all things (not **for** all things, but **in** all things). A thankful heart will open you up to receive from Him.

- Find something, **anything** to be thankful for! If you are in a constant state of negativity, it can hinder the ability of God's Word to work in your life.

MAKE IT YOUR OWN:

Lord, I thank You so much for everything You have done for me! You are an amazing God, and I am amazed at how wonderful You are to me! Thank You for sending Your Word to heal me and deliver me from all destruction. I am healed and delivered, in Jesus' name!

And the Word became flesh and dwelt among us, and we beheld His glory, the glory as of the only begotten of the Father, full of grace and truth.

› In order to really understand this verse, we need to go back to the first part of the book of John.

› John 1:1-3 – *¹ In the beginning was the Word, and the Word was with God, and the Word was God. ² He was in the beginning with God. ³ All things were made through Him, and without Him nothing was made that was made.*

› Jesus is the Word of God! **He *is* God**. When you read the Bible, you are hearing directly from Jesus. He is the Word of God who created the universe, who became a man for you.

› This is why there is so much power in the spoken Word of God! You are speaking that same creative power of Jesus into your life and circumstances!

MAKE IT YOUR OWN:

Lord Jesus, I understand that You are the Word of God made flesh. Thank You that when I speak Your Word over my life, my words have creative power!

10 For as the rain comes down, and the snow from heaven, And do not return there, But water the earth, And make it bring forth and bud, That it may give seed to the sower And bread to the eater, 11 So shall My word be that goes forth from My mouth; It shall not return to Me void, But it shall accomplish what I please, And it shall prosper in the thing for which I sent it.

- Jesus did not return to the Father void! He became a man and accomplished His purpose at the cross. That is why He said, *"It is finished."*

- When Jesus ascended back into Heaven, His work was complete! He finished everything that He was sent to accomplish.

- The Word of God does not return without accomplishing its purpose. When you speak the Word over your life, it is effective!

MAKE IT YOUR OWN:

Praise God! When I speak the Word over my life, it does not return void: it accomplishes its purpose. As I speak God's Word, it is effective in my life, bearing much fruit. I have whatever I say, in Jesus' name! Thank You, Lord, for this incredible gift of Your Word!

How God anointed Jesus of Nazareth with the Holy Spirit and with power, who went about doing good and healing all who were oppressed by the devil, for God was with Him.

- Jesus was anointed with the Holy Spirit and power, and He healed ALL!!

- This scripture indicates that anything that requires healing is an oppression of the devil. Now, this doesn't mean that the devil is personally attacking you every single time you become ill. However, the devil is the "god of this world" (2 Corinthians 4:4).

- Notice that in 2 Corinthians 4:4, the "god of this world" is a lowercase "g"! The devil has no power and authority that is greater than the power and authority that Jesus had, which He has given to you! (See Luke 10:19, page 23.)

MAKE IT YOUR OWN:

Thank You, Lord, that You are with me, just like You were with Jesus! I am anointed with the Holy Spirit and with power. I believe that I do good and heal all those who are oppressed by the devil, for You are with me, in Jesus' name.

² And behold, a leper came and worshiped Him, saying, "Lord, if You are willing, You can make me clean." ³ Then Jesus put out His hand and touched him, saying, "I am willing; be cleansed." Immediately his leprosy was cleansed.

- There is never an example in the Bible where someone came to Jesus for healing and He said, "No." There is also never a time when Jesus ever put sickness on someone to teach them a lesson.

- Jesus is **always** willing to heal! That is why He went to the cross and bore every sickness and disease. (See Isaiah 53:4-5 ; 1 Peter 2:24, pages 3-5.)

MAKE IT YOUR OWN:

Thank You, Jesus, that when I come to you for healing, You are willing! I believe that You want me well. Lord, help me to receive this healing that You have already provided for me. I receive my healing by faith right now, and I give thanks for it, in Jesus' name!

...For I am the Lord who heals you.

- The Lord is revealing to you His identity as your healer.

- God isn't just someone who heals. "Healer" is who He is! His nature is to heal you, not to make you sick.

MAKE IT YOUR OWN:

Lord, I believe that You are my Healer! Your very nature and identity is to heal me. I don't have to beg You to heal my body, because Your character is to heal, and You have been that way from the very beginning. You sent Jesus to provide healing to me, and I receive that healing by faith! I am a child of the Healer, and I am healed, in Jesus' name!

16 When evening had come, they brought to Him many who were demon-possessed. And He cast out the spirits with a word, and healed all who were sick, **17** that it might be fulfilled which was spoken by Isaiah the prophet, saying: "He Himself took our infirmities And bore our sicknesses."

- This verse makes an undeniable connection to Isaiah 53:4, that the prophet was writing about the Messiah providing physical healing for us on the cross.

- Notice that Jesus healed ALL who were sick. He taught them about the Kingdom of God, and then He healed them all. (Luke 4:40; Luke 9:11; Matt. 12:15).

- There is not one verse in the New Testament that speaks of an instance where someone came to Jesus for healing and He did not heal them.

MAKE IT YOUR OWN:

Jesus, I thank You for taking all of my sicknesses and pains on the cross. I can see by all of these scriptures that it is Your will for me to be well. And I know that if You healed all of them, You have healed me, too!

30 Then great multitudes came to Him, having with them the lame, blind, mute, maimed, and many others, and they laid them down at Jesus' feet, and He healed them. 31 So the multitude marveled when they saw the mute speaking, the maimed made whole, the lame walking, and the blind seeing; and they glorified the God of Israel.

- Look at all of these conditions that people had, yet Jesus healed them all. There is no condition that Jesus cannot heal and restore.

- The word for "lame" is *chólos,* which is "lame, deprived of a foot, limping". Jesus even healed those who were missing limbs!

- When Jesus heals, God is glorified!

MAKE IT YOUR OWN:

Lord, I thank you that there is no sickness, disease, or injury that is too hard for you to heal! I thank You for my healing, and I give you all the glory for it. I praise you for healing my body, in Jesus' name!

Wherever He entered, into villages, cities, or the country, they laid the sick in the marketplaces, and begged Him that they might just touch the hem of His garment. And as many as touched Him were made well.

- This verse is reminiscent of the story of the woman with the issue of blood who pressed through the crowd to touch the hem of His garment (Mark 5:25-34).

- Before the woman with the issue of blood, no one had every been healed that way before! Yet, after she believed, many others received their healing in the same way.

You can also follow their example! You definitely don't have to beg Him: He has already provided healing for you! However, you can reach out and receive it by faith, just like they did.

MAKE IT YOUR OWN:

Jesus, I thank You that you have made it a simple thing to receive healing from You. I believe You have provided healing for me at the cross, and I reach out and receive it by faith, right now! I am healed, in Jesus' name!

And the whole multitude sought to touch Him, for power went out from Him and healed them all.

- People could simply touch Jesus and the power inside of Him would heal them.

- Just like the woman with the issue of blood, if you will press in to Jesus, His power will make you whole.

- Today, it isn't the physical touch that brings healing. That is a representation of our faith in what Jesus has already done. The way we "touch" Jesus is through receiving by faith the power that He has freely provided to us. (See Romans 8:11, page 16.)

MAKE IT YOUR OWN:

Jesus, I may not be able to physically touch You, but what You have given me is even greater! The same Spirit who raised You from the dead lives in me and gives life to my body! I thank You for Your healing power that is flowing through me right now, from the inside out, in Jesus' name.

Jesus Christ is the same yesterday, today, and forever.

› Jesus has not changed. His will to heal when He walked the earth is no different than His will to heal today!

› The same God who created us never indended for us to even deal with sickness to begin with! He has not changed His mind about wanting us to live in health.

› You never have to question God's motives because He never changes! His steadfast faithfulness makes trusting Him very simple.

MAKE IT YOUR OWN:

Jesus, I believe Your Word, and it says that You will never change. I thank You that You want me well, and that You have provided that healing to me. I am healed, in Jesus' name!

Christ has redeemed us from the curse of the law, having become a curse for us (for it is written, "Cursed is everyone who hangs on a tree").

○ Throughout the Old Testament, you will read promises of God that are attached to a condition of behavior

○ Because of this, many modern believers disqualify themselves from receiving these promises because they can clearly see that they have not diligently obeyed God, nor carefully observed all of His commandments. They see the imperfection in their flesh and think they haven't earned these promises, and likely deserve the curses, too!

○ However, we can see here that Jesus redeemed us from the curses set forth in the law in Deuteronomy. Not only that, but Jesus actually perfectly fulfilled all of the requirements of the law *for us* so that we are not in bondage to that impossible standard of perfection. (Read Romans 8:3-4.)

○ 2 Corinthians 5:21 says that Jesus *became sin* so that you could be made righteous! Since you are a born-again believer, you *are* righteous. Therefore, you qualify for every single promise in the Old Testament, even the conditional ones! Jesus fulfilled all of those conditions for you.

MAKE IT YOUR OWN:

I am the righteousness of God in Christ Jesus. Jesus became the curse for me, so that I can live blessed. I realize that my righteousness is not based on my own perfect behavior, but on the perfection of Jesus. Thank You, Lord, that every single promised blessing in Your Word is mine, and that I have also been redeemed from every curse! Hallelujah!

- ○ (For more revelation regarding the curses that Jesus has redeemed you from, we encourage you to read Deuteronomy 28:16-68. You will be inspired when you confirm all of the curses that you are free from, including tumors, pests, defeat, lack, long-term illnesses, and so much more! Read that passage, and let the Holy Spirit reveal to you how complete your redemption is!)

25 So you shall serve the Lord your God, and He will bless your bread and your water. And I will take sickness away from the midst of you. 26 No one shall suffer miscarriage or be barren in your land; I will fulfill the number of your days.

- These blessings belong to you!

- God has promised to take sickness away from you.

- This is a particularly powerful verse for women who have experienced miscarriage, who are afraid of miscarriage, or who have had difficulty conceiving children. God says, "You will not suffer miscarriage and you are not barren! Be fruitful and multiply!"

- This promise is also one of a long, fulfilled life! It is not a blessing to die young. Jesus has redeemed you from that curse, and promises to fulfill your days

MAKE IT YOUR OWN:

Lord, thank You for blessing my food and water, and for taking sickness away from me. I will not suffer miscarriage or be barren. The fruit of my womb is blessed (Deuteronomy 28:4, 11), and I will live a fulfilled life, in Jesus' name!

Moses was one hundred and twenty years old when he died. His eyes were not dim nor his natural vigor diminished.

- This is an example of that fulfilled life! Moses was "old" when he died. But his eyesight was clear, and he was just as strong as he ever had been!

- Yes, we will all die someday, but we don't have to die sick and weak! Moses was strong enough to climb a mountain to die (and it wasn't the climb that killed him)! It was simply time for Joshua to lead the children of Israel into the Promised Land.

- When your purpose on this earth is complete, you can go home to be with Jesus. But that will only be when He has fulfilled the number of your days, no sooner.

- Hebrews 8:6 says, *"But in fact the ministry Jesus has received is as superior to theirs as the covenant of which he is mediator is superior to the old one, since the new covenant is established on **better promises** (NIV, emphasis added)."*

MAKE IT YOUR OWN:

I reject the lie that my body has to get painful, weak and sick before I die. I have a better covenant with God, based on better promises, than Moses did. Therefore, as I age, my eyesight is clear, my body is strong, and I will not die until I am ready, when I have fulfilled the number of my days! Thank You, Jesus, for a long, strong, healthy, fulfilled life!

I call heaven and earth as witnesses today against you, that I have set before you life and death, blessing and cursing; therefore choose life, that both you and your descendants may live.

> **God has given us a multiple choice test here, and then given us the answer!**

> The truth is, abundant life is a choice. You can choose death, through your thoughts, words and actions, or you can choose life with the same!

> If you will believe the Word of God and receive God's promises in your life through faith, you can overcome any challenge you face.

MAKE IT YOUR OWN:

choose life! I choose the truth in the Word of God, and I reject the lies of the enemy and the world. Holy Spirit, show me how I can choose life every day, in my thoughts, words and actions, in Jesus' name.

Fear not, for I am with you; Be not dismayed, for I am your God. I will strengthen you, Yes, I will help you, I will uphold you with My righteous right hand.

- Do not be afraid! God is faithful to fulfill His promises to you, so there is nothing for you to fear.

- All of His promises are "Yes"! (2 Corinthians 1:20). Yes, He will help you, He will strengthen you and He will hold You up!

- 2 Timothy 1:7 says that you have a spirit of power, love and a sound mind, not a spirit of fear.

- 1 John 4:18 tells us that perfect love casts out all fear. When you understand how much God loves you, you will never be afraid. You will know beyond a shadow of a doubt that God will never let you down!

MAKE IT YOUR OWN:

God has not given me a spirit of fear, but of power, love and a sound mind! I know the love of God for me, and it casts out all fear in my life. No matter what is going on, I am confident in His love for me and His faithfulness to fulfill all of His promises to me. He is strengthening me, helping me, and upholding me in His right hand!